THE NATURAL
HAIR BIBLE

Everything You Need to Know to
Grow Your Hair - Naturally

Dedication

This book is dedicated to my mother who taught me to take pride in my hair by meticulously caring for it every Sunday without fail until January 29, 2001. May God Continue to Rest Her Soul

INTRODUCTION

My name is Ashley and I'm pretty much obsessed with natural hair. So, I decided to write a book about it. This book was created for anyone who wants to be empowered to grow their hair —naturally; men, women, and even children. Although the information found in this book *does* cater more specifically to people of color, everyone can benefit from the knowledge of successfully and efficiently caring for their natural hair. Regardless of how you *choose* to wear your natural hair, whether that be with locs, braids, twist-outs, a silk press, a fade, high-top, wet n' wavy, or weaves; healthy hair needs proper care.

There are so many resources available today that we can utilize when educating ourselves about growing our hair in a healthy manner, but with the options seeming endless, where do we start? In a world of YouTube bloggers, Instagram hair gurus, popular natural haircare products, celebrities posting ads on social media of themselves using haircare products—where do we even begin with narrowing down all of the information into one easy and concise resource? Whose advice is best? Who can we trust? What works? Which products are gimmicks? I don't know about you but throughout my natural hair journey, I've tried numerous methods, made more mistakes than I can count, and have spent countless dollars purchasing product after product thinking it was going to somehow be a game-changer for me in my everyday hair routine.

I've been natural for the last seven years and the last five have been a sweet spot for me—mostly a pretty smooth-sailing venture for me as a result of all of the mistakes I've made in the past. Consequently, I've documented a natural routine for healthy, natural hair that can be implemented on any natural hair type. The coolest thing is, this routine is quite simple and involves products you may already have in your home. Once you're aware of the natural ingredients your hair needs for optimal growth, selecting the right hair product for your unique natural texture will become second nature. Together, we'll explore how to make the most of what you already have in your cabinets while ensuring your future purchases are the best choices for your natural hair. This book will cover specific tips and tricks for you to grow your best head of hair—while keeping it as natural as you can.

You and I will even review what a couple of hair experts had to say, and they spilled all the natural haircare tea about what's effective and what's not! Yes, finally...the TRUTH!

Speaking of the truth, caring for your natural hair is likely much simpler than you think. **It first begins with changing your mindset.** If you and I take the time to brush our teeth, moisturize our skin, shave our scruff, exfoliate our skin, and go to the gym; why wouldn't we make the time to properly care for our hair in an effort to grow it healthier? Come on; let's talk natural hair...

Table of Contents

CHAPTER 1: IN THE BEGINNING | HISTORY OF NATURAL HAIR

Natural: hair that is relaxer-free. You know, free from the creamy-crack.

In the Beginning...

I haven't always liked my hair. When I was in elementary school, I remember an older boy who insisted on teasing me about my pigtails that my mom would so carefully braid on my head in twos. Once upon a time, it was my favorite hairstyle. Yet, as I grew older, I began to feel self-conscious about my hair. It was thick, super curly and could get frizzy on the right Georgia day. I oftentimes wonder if that bully even has hair himself today...

It is estimated that between 1525 and 1866, some 12 million Africans were shipped via The Middle Passage to The New World. The majority of Africans, those who survived, were dropped off in South America and in the Caribbean. A small percentage, "only" approximately 388,000 were brought to North America. Many scholars estimate that after landing in the Caribbean, another 60,000 Africans ended up in the United States.

So, that puts us at about 450,000 that ended up here in the U.S. Think about how small that number actually is. There are approximately 327 million people in America right now. Those of us who mark "Black" or "African American" on the census survey make up about 13.4% of that population. So, with the exception of immigrants, there are roughly 42 million black Americans in the United States who are mostly derived from a group of Africans who were less than half a million in number.

I can only imagine how it was post-emancipation. Picture this: slavery was now illegal, but society still shunned you. Confusion about where to go, who to trust, where your family ended up, where your true heritage originated from. Self-image issues brought on by hundreds of years of damaging language that was intended to promote divisiveness and self-hatred still lingered inside many newly-freed blacks. Years of white plantation owners raping black female slaves resulting in them giving birth to biracial enslaved children provided a way for a new breed of loss identity that entered into the start of early Black American culture: **Colorism**. See, lighter skin tones wasn't *necessarily* something our early ancestors *wanted*, it was oftentimes viewed as something needed to survive. European features were more favored by plantation owners, consequently delivering lesser workloads to biracial slaves.

Nappy: one of the terms used to divide Blacks from *mulatto* children; both of whom were enslaved. In 2005, an underground-independent documentary hit the scene and it explored the term "Nappy." *My Nappy Roots: A Journey Through Black Hairitage*, educated us that Nap was a term exclusive to black slaves who worked in the cotton fields. Slave masters would refer to slaves' hair as being similar to the tuft of cotton that forms during the harvesting season called a nap. This is the only paragraph where the word nappy will be mentioned within *The Natural Hair Bible*. I understand many naturals have embraced the term, however, *The Natural Hair Bible* does not believe that to be a term of endearment when describing our hair.

Consider this: during slave auctions, biracial slaves were often sold at a higher price than their non-mixed counterparts. What type of mental consequences do you think were incurred as a result of this, if any? Is it possible our social perceptions surrounding color and hair within the black community are direct results from all those years of disparity? If so, how deep does the damage go?

Post emancipation, many blacks felt pressured to conform to European standards of beauty and would use chemicals to straighten their hair, even at the expense of sometimes burning their scalp. In the 1960s, amidst Civil Rights movements starting to increase, the Afro took off. It was to be worn with pride while representing freedom and rebellion simultaneously.

Today, black women wear their hair in a variety of styles including lacefront wigs, braids, sew-ins, locs, shaved off and more. Why? Because we can. Our hair is a versatile palette awaiting the right mold. Our hair is also delicate and in need of the proper routine and ingredients for prolonged health.

That's just a quick snippet of just how our natural hair journey has looked over the decades. We won't dive too much deeper, but I encourage you to do to more research about the journey our hair has taken since our ancestors arrived here. That's enough historical talk—we've got hair to do...

Learn Your Lingo

It's important to understand the terminology within the natural hair community so you can feel empowered when it comes to discussing methods with other naturals as well as understanding which methods work best for your hair.

Right now, you should flip to the back of the book and read through the terms located in the Natural Hair Glossary. Familiarize yourself with the natural hair slang and really take the time to analyze the definitions before we get started. Go ahead, I'll wait here.

Proceed to Chapter 2 once you're done.

CHAPTER 2: PRODUCTS EVERY NATURAL SHOULD HAVE

Styling Tools

I do believe there are specific styling tools every natural should have. I mean, they were invented to make our lives easier. Whether it's to try out a new style, maintain the current style, or to be used in daily maintenance; there are tools we should have within our personal arsenal. The funny thing is: you likely already have them.

Satin Pillowcase/Bonnet or Scarf

I ordered mine from Amazon, but these are sold at most general stores like Walmart or Sally's. These items are basics. You have to go to sleep right? Well, you definitely need the silk duo to ensure that: 1. Your hair stays properly moisturized (cotton sheets/pillowcases can cause intense drying of our hair) and 2. Your current style stays maintained. Whether your hair is in a **Twist Set** or simply in a bun on top of your head, satin is key.

Small Spray Bottle

The spray bottle is likely the cheapest tool on this list, but it is a powerful apparatus in the natural haircare routine. You can literally purchase them for $1 in the travel section of many all-purpose stores. I use my spray bottle several times each week and I know many naturals who use it daily. What's in it? Oh, your filtered water, of course, mixed with all of your favorite oils inside. Or, maybe you've got two spray bottles in rotation with the second being filled with your homemade rice water. I have one spray bottle that I switch out every few months (because you know, water mildews). I keep it in the refrigerator filled with my rice water. Don't get too caught up on the mention of the oil + water and rice water concoctions. We'll get to those details later.

Hairpins (as a natural, you need a lot of these)

Spare yourself from the heartache of losing your precious strands to some cheap hairpins. Get the good kind, keep a lot, and don't be afraid to use them. Whether hairpins are being used for buns, ponytails, bantu knots, or even a way to add a decorative style your normal everyday hairstyle, hairpins are a natural's go-to styling tool.

Ponytail Holders (all elastic, no metal)

So, I don't wear a lot of ponytails, but I use them often when I'm in the gym in an attempt to maintain my Twist Outs. Make sure that when you buy ponytail holders, you're not skimping on quality and buying the ones with metal on them. Why do they even make those anyway? Metal-LESS ponytails are the only way naturals should go!

[Insert your favorite] Oil

Coconut oil is my hair's favorite oil. We'll cover the major oils for naturals later in the book. For now, just know you need at least one staple oil for your regimen.

Flexi-rods

Flexi-rods are long, bendable styling tools with a metal wire down the center. They are sold in different rod colors which indicates their curl width. They're some of my favorite styling tools because they are a "set-n-go" type of styling tool. The downside is sleeping in them. Nevertheless, I like to use flexi-rods during the holidays and I experiment with the different widths to create various styles. Flexi-rods are also a great way to re-vamp your midweek hairstyle on an older Twist or Braid Out.

Perm-rods

Overall, I enjoy using flexi-rods more because they're so easy to install, however, perm rods have a place in my natural haircare regimen, too. I use perm-rods at the ends of my hair when I do Twist-Outs to accentuate an even curl throughout. They can even be used to emulate a blowout if you use the larger sizes. Many naturals have amazing results with perm rods.

My Favorite Styling Products

In my college years, I was a **Product Junkie,** but throughout the last few years, my main focus has been finding the right *natural ingredients* to be used on my hair. This chapter is the only time you'll see name brands mentioned as examples in *The Natural Hair Bible* (NHB). The focus of the book is on specific natural ingredients that are best for our hair; not specific product brands. However, I do have my preferences favoring a few major products currently on the market that I'd like to share as they've been very key for me in reaching my natural hair goals:

Shampoo Favorites

These are my favorites because they are mild and get the job done; which is cleansing my scalp. As you will read later in the book, I don't shampoo my hair often enough to have several favorites. If I notice my hair/scalp is dirtier than usual, I'll use **Option 1**. If I just want to cleanse my hair with no actual problem areas in mind, I'll use **Option 2** as it has fantastic fatty emollients in it that moisturize the hair as it cleanses.

Option 1: Trader Joe's Tea Tree Tingle Shampoo
Option 2: African Black Soap

Conditioner Favorites

These are my favorite conditioners because they provide loads of Slip when I am styling or detangling my hair. I'll use **Option 1** after a final conditioner when rinsing out a DC treatment. I use **Option 2** as a leave-in to be used a couple of times a week and immediately after applying coconut oil to my hair once my final rinse/wring is complete on **Wash Day**. Notice how I have a couple of normal to moderate conditioners as well as a couple of deeper penetrating masks on this below list:

Option 1: Trader Joe's Tea Tree Tingle Conditioner

Option 2: Manechoice 3-in-1 Leave-In Conditioner

Option 3: Manechoice Deep Strengthening & Restorative Mask Treatment

Option 4: Shea Moisture Deep Treatment Masque

Oil Favorites

Coconut Oil is the go-to oil that never fails me. We'll read more into the actual benefits of Coconut Oil as we explore the NHB deeper, but for now, just know this is my supreme choice of oil.

Option 1: Coconut Oil

Styling Favorites

I only have one true preferred styler as I tend to use my favorite natural hair oil in conjunction with my favorite leave-in conditioner to style my hair along with, of course, water. I use **Option 1** right before I begin styling my hair on **Wash Day**. I enjoy this styler because of its light scent, ability to seal moisture, and versatility with different natural hairstyles as I use it on Twist Outs and even Flexi-rod sets.

Option 1: Manechoice Doesn't get much Butter Than This.

CHAPTER 3: DANGER: STAY AWAY

There are several practices that naturals should stay away from IF they are looking to consistently grow their hair in a natural and healthy way. Let's go through each one by one and explore why these methods aren't ideal.

Frequent Shampooing: We'll talk about this more in an upcoming chapter, but frequent shampooing can lead to dryness which causes breakage which leads to, well, you know, limited growth and retention. Learn to embrace and love conditioner. It's your best friend. When I tell people I wash my hair approximately every three months, I'm always served a look of either concern, disgust, or perplexity. What they aren't realizing is that I co-wash my hair weekly. This simply means I am "washing" it with conditioner instead. Over-shampooing our natural hair has costly implications. Our kinks and curls thrive off of natural oils so shampooing too frequently could cause unwanted breakage.

Frequent Application of Heat: So this one rattles people's cages and I get it. Just because you add heat to your hair, doesn't necessarily mean it's unhealthy. Just because you're natural, doesn't mean your hair is healthy either. Natural hair health can be recognized through, shine, elasticity, lack of split ends and breakage with a well moisturized hair shaft.

What matters is how you want to wear your hair and what looks good on you—to you. For instance, I like to wear my natural hair in its textured state, so I don't prefer a lot of heat application to my kinks and curls because it does have the ability to make our natural curl pattern uneven and inconsistent. Remember, your natural hair is trainable, so natural hair, over time, can be trained to have a more relaxed texture pattern if it's used to being constantly straightened. However, many naturals have told me that they don't mind a little heat damage and actually like it because it allows them to more easily wear their hair straight. See what I mean? It's all about how you enjoy wearing your hair and what your ultimate goals are.

Is your goal to grow long, luscious hair that you can wear in its natural state most of the time with a uniformed curl pattern throughout? Well then, you and frequent application of high heat may never see eye-to-eye. If you're not able to complete a safe silk-press yourself, it's important to find a trusted and educated natural haircare professional who can assess the appropriate amount of heat your hair can take without damaging its texture. Not all silk presses are created equal.

Frequent Combing
Frequent combing, especially on hair that is dry and/or brittle can lead to unnecessary hair breakage. I rarely use a comb unless it's a rattail comb for parting my hair to create sections. Finger detangling is a much more natural way of detangling because it allows you to work through areas of tangle with your fingers which allows for maximum hair retention.

Frequent Brushing
See aforementioned **Frequent Combing**. In addition, tough bristles overused on the nape or hairline can cause hair breakage.

Products with Sulfate...?
Well, well...it's the age-old controversial topic amongst naturals. Are sulfates good or bad? Healthy to use or damaging? Sulfates are the main reason why many products have great foaming abilities when cleansing hair. If you have naturally dry hair or hair that tends to become easily dried out, look for a sulfate-free cleanser. Although sulfates are SAFE to use, they can be very dry-

ing for certain natural hair types due to the stripping its agents cause on the hair after cleansing.

Many naturals with kinks and coils find sulfate cleansers to be quite drying and will notice frizz after washing. My hair doesn't like sulfate cleansers at all, which takes me to my next point. Know *your* hair. Just because my hair doesn't take well to sulfates doesn't mean yours can't benefit from it. Although essential oils are, for the most part, good for our hair, excessive oil can trap dirt and bacteria on the hair shaft and scalp. So, be sure to keep your eye out on the cleanliness of your hair when sulfates may be helpful for dirt removal.

Frequent Tension on the Hairline (Ponytails/Weaves/Buns/Braids)

The fact of the matter is: styles that are too tight can cause irreversible hair loss and damage. I know it may seem like the obvious but let's just break it down: when styles are sewn, braided, twisted, pulled, and/or secured too tightly for extended periods of time, Traction Alopecia can occur.

Excessive tension on your delicate hair follicles can lead to them being inflamed which can cause scaly skin around the tension-filled area. Prolonged tension can even cause pimple-like bumps to surround the area of inflamed hair follicles. Sometimes, people will experience hair loss on the nape of the neck, others in the center of their head and even more from the hairline surrounding their forehead and ears. If noticed early enough, this can be reversed. Permanent balding occurs when the issue has been ignored for too long.

Alcohols

FACT: Not all alcohols are created equal! That's right, I said it. They're not. As naturals, we must stay informed on all ingredients when it comes to our hair products. Remember, this book isn't about creating *more **Product Junkies***, rather, it's about serving as a resource for us naturals on what ingredients are used in the products around us and evaluating them for our personal hair usage.

Beware of Products that Contain These Alcohols:
- Ethanol
- Alcohol Denat
- Propanol
- Isopropyl
- Propyl
- SD Alcohol 40

Try Products with These Alcohols:
- Lauryl
- Cetyl
- Myristyl
- Behenyl
- Stearyl

What makes these alcohols better than the rest? These are fatty alcohols that are filled with emollient properties that can help create **Slip** in many of the products they're included in. Many of our favorite conditioners contain these good alcohols, so don't be afraid to use these.

CHAPTER 4: OKAY, NOW CURL THIS WAY

Now that we've discussed the practices and products that don't help us obtain our best head of natural hair, let's talk about what things we *should* be using or doing:

Finger Detangle

Finger detangling is one of the most effective ways for us to keep our natural hair free from tangles without tearing it all out. Your fingers are a lot more gentle than a comb when it comes to unraveling those infamous two-strand knots that naturals so often develop in their kinks and curls. For more information see Finger Detangling in the Natural Hair Glossary.

Protective Styles (find one that works best for you)

My favorite is the Twist-Out because it's quick and easy. In fact, I've been doing the same style for so many years now, my hair is trained to fall in the exact direction of how I always do my twist-out. That's the cool part about natural hair: it *can* be trained. Later in this book, we will explore other style ideas for naturals. For more details about how to perfect your twist-out, I suggest choosing one of the social media resources from Chapter 8.

Deep Conditioning (DC)

Deep conditioning is one of the most important steps in the natural haircare process, especially for those of us who live in dry climates. Deep conditioning allows you to be creative, too! I deep condition every Sunday and my hair enjoys trying different hot oils mixed into the conditioner. I encourage naturals to treat the DC process like a chemistry project. Start with your preferred conditioner and add the essentials whether it be hot oil, honey, or another natural resource to aid your hair back to a healthy moisturized state.

Use Water on the Hair for Proper Moisture

I think this step is commonly missed. Many naturals load their hair up with oil and other moisturizing products, missing the most important and only actual moisturizer there is: water. Due to worldwide water systems having inconsistent chemicals in them (Nitrate, Monochloramine, etc.), it's in our best interest to use filtered water when rinsing, washing, and dampening via a spray bottle. Try using filtered water for your next few washes and see if you feel a difference.

Cleanse the Scalp Periodically

Keeping a clean scalp is key to ensuring new growth has a clean environment to thrive. ACV is a fantastic resource for rinsing your scalp before or after co-washing. Keeping an eye *and* nose out on how your hair usually looks and smells is key. You know your hair better than anyone else. ACV is an anti-inflammation, antifungal product that has great benefits when used on the scalp. Don't forget the "big, bad" sulfates too. If you've got major build-up on your scalp, sulfates may be able to save the day.

Use Less Shampoo and More Conditioner

...because shampooing is overrated. No, but really—it is. Over the last few years, I've drastically minimized the number of times I shampoo my hair. As a result, I've been able to retain so much moisture in my hair. While it's important to keep your scalp clean, it's equally pertinent to keep your hair shaft and ends moisturized. Co-washing has become a weekly habit of mine. On average, I shampoo every 3-4 months. If you're co-washing each week and using naturally-based products, you shouldn't have to shampoo often since dirt, build-up, and bacteria will likely be minimal on your scalp.

Natural Concoctions for Hair Growth

Water/Oil Spray Mixture

You should be adding water to your hair frequently. If you aren't—look in the mirror. Is your hair dry? Remember, oil can do nothing for your natural hair without water mixed with it. Make sure you have a water/oil mixture for your hair that you use daily (at night). Add filtered water to a small spray bottle (no exact measurements, just eyeball it), add your oils: extra virgin olive oil, jojoba oil, black Jamaican castor oil, etc. Before spraying, shake the bottle some and lightly spritz. Be careful not to saturate the hair, just spray it lightly. If I'm just refreshing my style for the week, I don't spray too much as I don't want my hair to revert back (a.k.a. shrink) so, I just spray lightly.

Fermented Rice water

Rice water has essential nutrients such as Amino acids, B vitamins and Vitamin E. I originally started using rice water when I was searching for a natural way to prevent hair breakage while promoting hair growth. In my search, rice water came up. According to researchers, women in the Heian period (794 to 1185 CE) in Japan had floor-length hair they kept healthy by bathing it in rice water. Rice water has the unique ability to add shine, make hair smoother, promotes hair growth, detangles hair, and of course makes it stronger. For information on how to make rice water, visit YouTube!

Take Your Vitamins

Taking supplements daily that are natural with no synthetic dyes or fillers, although aren't a fix-all, have some benefits that could lead to an overall healthier state which of course improves your hair, skin, and nails. While multivitamins have been at the heart of controversy in regard to their usefulness and safety, do your research on which safe and helpful all-around multivitamin would be best for you. Scientifically speaking, eating a balanced diet with whole grains and vegetables being at the forefront can do a world of difference for your hair growth and health.

Exercise

As alluded to above, a healthy lifestyle is key for overall health which includes growing your best head of natural hair. Consistently exercising leads to better blood circulation within the body. Better blood circulation allows essentials nutrients and oxygen to reach your follicles, and consequently your follicles are more stimulated, which induces hair growth. Sweating also has the ability to help reveal dirt and other bacteria that maybe hiding out in your scalp.

Drink Water

While we're on the health kick, you knew this one was coming, right? Water and overall health are directly intertwined —we know this. When a body is dehydrated, one of the first physical signs may be dry, brittle hair. Ensuring your body is fully hydrated will help with a variety of other health concerns. Drink a lot of water. It's proven to cause hair to grow faster. It's said that our bodies are made up of about 60% water and that one hair strand is made up of about 25% water. Bottom line; ensure you're having a proper intake of water.

CHAPTER 5: WILL THE REAL NATURAL HAIR PRODUCTS PLEASE STAND UP?

The Natural Hair Bible is all about hair care and less about being a product snob or product junkie. Advertising specific hair-care brands is not the premise of this book. The empowerment lies within you. We've already covered which alcohols are better than others when searching for products to use on our hair. Let's dig deeper...

My overall hair product advice would be to find what works for your hair and utilize all of your resources. For instance, I use natural ingredients along with more popular hair products that include the natural ingredients that I like. See what I mean? Using high-quality, professionally sold hair products in conjunction with natural products is a game-changer. Oftentimes, your dry and brittle hair may need a truly formulated DC. We'll talk about this later in Chapter 8. I mean, really *find* what works. Pay attention to your tresses on a day-to-day basis. For me, I can feel when my hair is dryer than other times and when it appears to be more voluminous than other days. When you and I pay attention, we'll notice that our hair speaks volumes.

Keeping in mind the information you've already learned about which ingredients are best for your hair in terms of alcohol, let's get down to the Top Ingredients to look for when purchasing natural haircare products:

Water

Ahh, the greatest natural ingredient on Earth. Be sure to look for water as the first or main ingredient in your products. When you wash your hair, try to use filtered water. I try to think about water first before I do anything to my hair. It's important to have an oil-based sealing product that can be applied to your hair once you've *watered* it. Not following up with a high-quality sealant allows water to dry your natural hair out.

Honey

With its emollient and humectant properties, honey lends itself to adding moisture and overall scalp health amongst some of its main benefits of use for natural hair. Humectants are molecules that allow moisture to be retained. Honey isn't new on the block. It's been used for centuries in traditional medicine. In addition to honey being a natural antibacterial resource, its humectant properties bond with, you guessed it: water, in a successful effort in locking in moisture to our hair. Bottom line: PROTECT THE BEES! No, but seriously—natural hair loves honey. Honey can serve as a hair conditioner, a hair lightening agent, and even a preventative measure for hair loss or breakage.

Coconut Oil

Coconut oil is my sealant and miracle oil of choice. My hair loves its scalp-health abilities and its usefulness in adding shine as well as aiding in hair length and retention. We'll get into **Wash Day** later in the book but for now, just know that I put at least two handfuls of coconut oil onto my hair after my final rinse/wring while my hair is still wet. It keeps my hair moisturized throughout the week and allows me to easily finger detangle once mixed with my leave-in conditioner.

Avocado Oil

Avocados have a great source of monosaturated fats that

allow the hair to absorb and retain moisture. They also have a great source of Vitamins A, D, and E and are a good source of potassium as well. Avocado oil isn't as easy to find as coconut oil and other hair oils, but if you do come across it, consider adding it to your natural hair regimen.

Shea Butter

One of the natural resources our ancestors utilized prior to being shipped to the *New World* was shea butter. Hailing from Western Africa, shea butter nuts are grown on the Karite Tree. Shea butter is a great emollient that reduces the amount of water (moisture) lost from our natural hair. It's high in fatty acids and even has the ability to protect hair from the sun. Shea butter has several other beauty benefits that I encourage naturals to take advantage of. It is a natural antioxidant and contains Vitamins A and E along with essential fatty acids.

Tea Tree Oil

Tea tree oil is derived from a native tea tree shrub originating from Australia. The oil has the ability to rid fungus and microbes, making it a powerful antifungal, antibacterial resource that can be used on our natural hair. Having an excessively oily scalp or scalp plagued with dandruff can impede the new hair growth process, so ensuring your scalp is clean and healthy will assist you with reaching your natural haircare goals. I enjoy using tea tree tingle infused shampoo and conditioner when my scalp has felt more irritated than usual. You can typically feel tea tree opening up your hair follicles which provides a sensation that your scalp is *breathing*. Whether you like using tea tree oil by itself or infused in a product, there are several benefits to this natural resource.

Castor Oil

The humectant hype is totally real right now! Hear me when I say that oils that contain humectants don't necessarily *grow* your hair, rather, they allow your hair to retain moisture which leads to less hair breakage, and greater hair growth retention. Castor oil has the ability to penetrate deeper than other oils on this list—a word of advice for those naturals experiencing extreme dryness.

Aloe Vera

Aloe Vera has great slip that can aid in your detangling process by being mixed into your favorite conditioner or hair mask. It also helps with a variety of scalp disorders while unclogging your hair follicles from dirt and other bacteria. You can purchase Aloe Vera leaves at your local grocer.

Arrowroot Powder

With its origins coming all the way from South America, this natural resource has multiple benefits when it comes to our natural hair and even cooking. After the powder is extracted from the arrowroot plant, which can grow up to five feet tall, it goes through different stages before we are able to use it as a powder. After it has completed its liquid stage and dried in the sun, it forms a powder. It has the unique ability to absorb excess oil leaving the hair feeling silky and soft. I don't find this ingredient in too many natural hair products, but it's out there. Keep your eyes out for it.

Vegetable Glycerin

Remember humectants that we talked about with honey? Well, vegetable glycerin has humectants as well making it a great retainer of moisture. Products containing vegetable glycerin usually have great slip.

Jojoba Oil

The humectant molecule benefits continue with jojoba oil. I love jojoba oil because it isn't greasy feeling like other, heavier oils. It creates great shine as well!

EVOO (Extra Virgin Olive Oil)

This cooking oil is made without using any type of chemical. It has multiple softening emollients that make deep conditioning a lot more manageable. With no industrial refinement involved in the crushing process, EVOO has several other beauty benefits for the skin as well.

In Short...These natural ingredients can be used by themselves, mixed with one another, or added to other high-quality hair products. I encourage you to find which oils your hair loves and go from there. Keeping it simple and in reference to the LOC process, the basic items I use for my natural hair are: Water **(Liquid)** Coconut Oil **(Oil)** and 3-in-1 Leave-in Conditioner by Manechoice **(Cream)**. Have you developed your custom LOC process? Now that you're armed with the key ingredients you should look for in your natural haircare products, it's time for **Wash Day.**

CHAPTER 6:
WASH DAY

Growing up, I baked a lot with my mom. I reminisce about her cooking by remembering her amazing sweet potato pie, perfectly cooked rice, scrumptious black-eyed peas, and her simple yet amazing Rice Krispy Treats. She taught me the importance of setting the oven to the appropriate temperature, the difference of mixing and whisking, the taste differences between baking vs. boiling along with demonstrating the beauty of patience in order to get a perfectly baked result. Her lessons of heat temperatures and what materials to cover food with while baking (aluminum foil, parchment paper, etc.) remain fresh in my mind today and have relevancy to Wash Day for our natural hair.

Similarly to cooking, Wash Day has a few temperature changes, multiple ingredient mixtures, and a need for patience as the hair "bakes" and absorbs all ingredients that were so carefully added. Wash Day is a science that can be enhanced by the LOC method. It is the method I stand behind, which has been a staple in my natural haircare regimen for the last few years. **Below is my weekly Wash/Deep Conditioning routine:**

1. **Pre-poo**: This is the method by which the hair is prepped prior to washing, typically done with a conditioner and/or oil. Pre-pooing adds extra moisture to the hair and allows detangling to be much easier. You'll also be giving your hair a little extra lovin' for the oven.

    a. Use your spray bottle to dampen the hair with rice water (do not drench the hair in water). Apply conditioner with an oil mixture while sectioning hair and twisting, braiding, or bantu-knotting. However you decide to secure the hair while it is drenched with conditioner doesn't matter—the point is to have the hair sectioned and out of the way. During this step, I am finger detangling as I section and secure. If you feel you need a little more help with your hair, use a wide-toothed comb or our trusted friend: the Denman brush.

b. Apply a thin plastic shower cap (you know the ones that come in a pack of fifty) or regular grocery bag to your hair and allow to sit for at least twenty to thirty minutes. For extra added moisture —go to the gym! I know many of you thought I was going to say, "sit under the dryer." You can do that too! The point is to heat up your scalp and create humidity within the plastic cap. You can call this the homemade steam treatment.

2. **Shampoo/Co-Wash**: As you discovered earlier, I typically co-wash my hair weekly instead of shampooing. However, let's go through both methods together. I want to be sure you understand how they differ. Find which is best for your hair and do that.

a. **Shampoo**: After rinsing out your pre-poo, find your favorite moisturizing, possibly sulfate-free shampoo and focus on the roots of the hair. Attempt to purchase shampoos free of SLSs as it tends to dry our hair more than it helps. I hear many say that a clarifying shampoo is best, and then follow that up with a moisturizing shampoo. But if you're keeping your hair as natural as you can while using the process we've covered so far, rarely should you need a clarifying shampoo because your scalp should be pretty free of a large amount of residue buildup. Washing your hair in lukewarm water with your preferred shampoo is best.

b. **Co-Wash**: After rinsing out your pre-poo with lukewarm water, I typically apply another moisturizing conditioner that I enjoy and allow to sit in my hair for a few moments while in the shower. This is usually a good time for me to wash my face and exfoliate. Understand that you do not *have* to condition it for a second time, that's just an extra added step that I take to ensure my hair is fully moisturized—I've been in the desert for two years and my hair and the heat been in a one-on-one battle since. The last step: rinsing with a cold bottle of water. Unless your water can be proven to be without many unnatural chemicals that are typically found in tap water, it's best to use filtered or bottled water for the extra shine and softness. Having a cool rinse at the end of your conditioning sessions leaves a positive effect on your hair as it helps close the cuticles and pores while increasing the shine.

3. **Post Wash**

After the final cool rinse has been completed, I wring my hair out with my hands. I then take a couple of handfuls of coconut oil and apply liberally throughout my hair while still in the shower. Once completed, I wrap my hair in a T-shirt to get rid of the excess water, apply my leave-in conditioner, and begin to style.

CHAPTER 7: STYLIN' N PROFILIN'

The idea of unique hairstyles within the black community has been around since early African civilization. Then, hairstyles oftentimes indicated a person's family background, tribe, and social status. Elaborate hairstyles were a deep segment of the West African culture. Once our ancestors were shipped from Africa to the *New World,* their hair was cut off—a first step in eradicating identity and culture.

If we go back *To the Beginning,* we'll be reminded that our ancestors were taken away from their natural resources (shea butter and the like) which they used to care for their hair pre-Transatlantic Slave Trade. Consequently, they had to become creative with the resources they used for their hair. With resources limited to them, chemicals like kerosene and lubricants like butter were used to moisturize their hair. During the years leading up to the abolishment of slavery and thereafter, blacks used other chemicals like lye mixed with potato, which was used to straighten natural hair in an effort to keep up with European beauty standards.

There are a few styles that every natural can benefit from mastering. For me, I'm still trying to learn how to braid. I know, I know...I should totally know how to braid, but I don't. Plaiting? Oh, I've got that down to a science. It's the whole, adding hair thing that gets me. I'll learn that skill one day—especially before I, prayerfully, have a daughter.

Twist-Out

The Twist-Out is my go-to hairstyle. It's what I wear on a daily and weekly basis and can be styled down, up, in a bun, in pigtails, half up and half down, and so many more ways. I love this style because when done well, it lasts the entire week. This style is easily preserved during a workout as well, which for me, is key. I don't like when my hairstyle impedes my ability to be physically active. Oftentimes, if I want my twist-out to be more defined during the week, I'll lightly spray with water and loosely re-twist with my favorite hair pomade or leave-in conditioner. I get my best twist-outs when I follow the LOC method and carefully flat twist the hair which creates uniformed sections of curls and coils that can be pulled apart throughout the week.

WnGs

A wash-and-go can be a naturals' worst nightmare. For others, it's a saving grace. For me, it depends on the climate I'm currently in. During 2014, I worked in Austin, Texas for six months. The weather was extremely humid and hot during the summer. I wore WnGs almost daily. I'd wet my hair with water and add my favorite leave-in-conditioner and a leave-in styler and go. Sometimes, if I wanted a less-wet look, I'd use my diffuser on the cool setting immediately after applying my styler. My hair was well moisturized and I had lots of volume.

I currently live in the dry desert of Las Vegas. Some may think this is the perfect weather for wearing WnGs, but for my hair, this extremely dry climate does not allow my best WnGs to occur. Much of our natural hair journey relies on us learning what our hair likes and what it doesn't. For a great wash-and-go, I encourage naturals to make leave-in conditioner their best friend. When applying a leave-in after you've wet the hair in water, it helps prevent tangles and allows your coils and curls to be shown in their natural beauty without knots. My curls *love* to kink up in two-strand knots, so for me, leave-in conditioner is required.

Once, I had to cut off four inches of hair due to my hair drying out and becoming brittle while working in Denver, Colorado for six months as I was doing WnGs a few times each week. Not only was I not applying a creamy leave-in conditioner immediately after saturating my hair, I wasn't applying an oil either. I didn't realize the gel I was applying after I was getting out the shower contained no humectants and a couple of drying alcohols, which left my hair dry, brittle and breaking off as a result of too many WnGs done incorrectly.

Braid-outs

As I mentioned earlier, I'm still learning how to braid, but... that doesn't mean I'm completely out of the game! Oftentimes, after washing my hair, I'll braid it in four large plaits and allow it to air dry. This gives me a different look with my hair that tends to be a little more stretched out than a twist-out. Braid-outs can be maintained similarly to twist-outs by applying a silk scarf at night. My favorite way to maintain my natural hairstyles in the evening before bed is with my hair in a pineapple covered by a silk scarf.

Low-tension buns

Buns are also another favorite of mine. High buns, low buns, midway buns, any bun is my favorite—as long as it is low tension. Low tension meaning, it isn't pulling on the nape of your hairline or edges as a result of being tight. Buns offer a sleek look that can be dressed up or down, worn to the boardroom or gym—it's all about finding the right bun for your head shape and your hair texture. There are times I wear my hair in the same bun all week! It's a great protective style that involves low-manipulation, which tends to look better with time.

Flexi-rods

I enjoy using flexi-rods to refresh and reconstruct a style like an old twist-out or to create a nice uniformed set of curls after co-washing the hair. During the holiday season, I oftentimes do this hairstyle as it can dress up your normal day-to-day hairstyle. Using the exact same co-washing method and post-wash products you'd use on your twist-out, install flexi-rods instead of doing your usual twist-out or braid-out.

Stretching

Look up the banding method in the back of this book in the Natural Hair Glossary for an example of stretching. Stretching isn't really a style per se, more like a method by which to prep the next style in lieu of re-washing the hair. If you've been wearing a twist-out all week and want a different look to finish out the week or to prepare for the next week's style without washing, consider stretching the hair to: imitate a blowout, allow easier prepping for updos and create different looking ponytails and buns and so much more. Oftentimes, if you've worn your hair in the same ponytail or bun for the entire week, the hair is likely already in a stretched out manner from being pulled back.

CHAPTER 8: RELIABLE RESOURCES

This book is called *The Natural Hair Bible* because it is all-encompassing. Its purpose is to serve as a resource to naturals everywhere. With so many "experts" in today's society who all claim to know about natural hair and what works, it can oftentimes be confusing. I have a selected few whom I go to for natural hair advice because they've been tried and true. Trusted and affirmed. Knowledgeable and educated.

Social Media Favorites

@Naptural85- Whitney White

I've been following Whitney since she first started her natural haircare videos on YouTube in 2009. She has over 1 million subscribers on her YouTube channel and has still managed to, "keep it real." She never straightens her hair by way of silk pressing and offers many creative alternatives for styling and caring for your natural hair including using actual natural haircare products like flaxseed gel and shea butter. She inspired me to start using flaxseed gel early on in my natural haircare journey. I also learned how to two-strand twist watching Whitney, which completely changed the "natural hair game" for me.

@MahoganyCurls - Jessica Lewis

Jessica is one of my favorite natural haircare bloggers because she continues to reinvent herself! She's done several BCs after having tons of length on her naturally curly tresses. I tried Curlformers for the first time after watching Jessica's tutorials on

YouTube. Although I no longer use Curlformers, it allowed me to start thinking outside of the box when it came to my natural curls and to see my hair as a versatile blank slate. I enjoy Jessica's tutorials because when she had longer hair, she was much like me with wearing her natural curls somewhat the same way every day. She is very good at maintaining her curls day-by-day and my "pineapple" method was perfected after watching her videos on maintaining her twist-outs.

@Curldaze - Robyn

Out of the three bloggers, Robyn's hair texture is most like mine which makes it easier for me to follow her tutorials. She has perfected the WnG method and has allowed me to perfect my flexi-rod method for a different look on my natural hair that can be more dressed up than my day-to-day twist-out look. She has a lot of fun with her hair and uses gels, buns, braids, and twists to put a spin on her everyday hairstyles.

Experts Weigh In

When YouTube and Instagram aren't enough and I need expert advice, I have two experienced natural haircare experts that have cared for my hair for a total of ten years between the two. They are each top caliber in the natural hair community and I've referred several people to them throughout the years. They have graciously given their time and educated advice for the readers of this book. I asked them key questions that naturals want to know and each have given their feedback. Their salon and booking information can also be found below for those readers who would like to have a consultation and styling appointment with them. Let's begin.

Nikk Nelson started doing my hair when I was only seventeen years old. I came to him with a head full of hair that was matted in so many areas. My hair was curly, thick, and frizzy! My late mother's best friend, Valerie (God rest both of their souls) took me to N'Seya Salon on Roswell Road in Sandy Springs, Georgia when I was just a teen. Nikk Nelson was the stylist who took my appointment that day. He saved my hair by cutting all eighteen inches off to just past my ears. I also wanted a perm and although he didn't think I needed one, it would help me care for my hair properly at that time when I was unknowledgeable about my natural haircare. My hair grew out to my shoulders within eight months. I continued going to Nikk all throughout college where he allowed me to experience some "firsts" with my hair. My first perm, my first blunt cut with straight bangs, my first hair shows, my first hair photoshoot and more.

Today, Nikk is a much sought-after celebrity stylist whose work has been seen on: Oscar winner Ruth Carter, Angela Simmons, Vanessa Simmons, Jeanette Jenkins, Tasha Smith, Terri J. Vaughn, Teyana Taylor, Christina Millian and many more. His work has also been featured on shows such as 106 & Park, The Game, America's Got Talent, Rip the Runway and Real Housewives of Atlanta just to name a few. He is a master stylist who is also a hair restoration specialist for people experiencing hair loss. Now that you know a bit about Nikk, let's see what he had to say about Natural Hair:

What is the most common myth regarding natural haircare that you hear from your clients?

The most common myth that I hear from clients is that in order to go from relaxed to natural, you have to cut all of the relaxed part off. You don't. In actuality, relaxed hair can make the transition for some a little easier. It allows you to maintain straight hair while training the new natural hair.

How can weave be worn as a protective style without it damaging the real hair underneath? Any tips on how frequently one would need it maintained?

Weaves can definitely be worn to protect the natural hair and grow the hair as well. You want to make sure your stylist is a reputable one in the industry first and foremost. Extensions are a luxury service and going the discounted route will most times not be the best option in the long run. You want to make sure to start with clean, conditioned hair and ensure your foundation or braid down is sturdy but not tight. You should always use netting because it protects the natural hair. When stitching, stitch into the net. You should get your extensions maintained just like you would your natural hair, every week or two. You shouldn't keep extensions any longer than 2 ½ to 3 months. Lastly, ALWAYS see a professional to remove your extensions.

What are your top 3 tips you give to your clients regarding caring for their natural hair?

My top 3 tips are:

1. *See your stylist regularly. You should see your stylist twice a month, especially if you are pressing your hair.*

2. *Ensure your natural hair has a hydration/steam treatment. It's the best way to add moisture and shine.*

3. *Understand that everyone's hair is different, so products are not a one size fits all type of thing. You should shop around for hair products that work well with your hair and texture. With the amount of natural hair products on the market now, you're sure to find your perfect match.*

Is there ONE product you feel like changed the natural hair game?

The one product that I feel changed the hair game is the Amino Smoothing System. In my experience, everyone that wants to be relaxer-free may not necessarily want to be the coiled and curled type of natural. Some may still want to maintain the straight or PRESSED look. The smoothing system allows for straight hair without the harshness of a relaxer and you can also still wear the natural texture of your hair as well. So, it's extremely versatile which is what most women want.

How can men ensure their natural hair is also kept healthy? Any general styling tips or specific detail when it comes to haircuts?

The thing is, hair is hair: whether it's on a male or female. The regimen that women use for natural hair can pretty much be used across the board. I have male clients that come in for shampoo and steam conditioners before their haircuts and I use some of the same products on them as I do on my female clients. Men these days take care of their hair just as much as women.

Nikk Nelson
Pressed Natural Hair Care
644 Antone Street NW #5
Atlanta, Georgia 30318
https://www.pressedhair.com/

Next up, we've got Monique:

Monique offered her expert advice on the same questions that were asked of Nikk. She has several hundred clients and usually books out months in advance. She has been doing my hair for the last five years and has been with me through several hair changes including my first highlights, cold weather damage that required me to cut three to four inches off (thanks, Denver!), my first set of braids, and more. She is a trusted professional whom I adore and I've sent several people her way throughout the years.

What I like about Monique is that she takes her time and cares for every single strand—individually. She is extremely knowledgeable about daily haircare products and encourages the use of high-quality professional products in conjunction with natural ingredients and treatments when I am doing my own hair. The combination of the high-quality products she uses on my hair in combination of the natural treatments like deep conditioning and rice-water have really allowed my hair to flourish.

She is a licensed master Hairstylist and color specialist of thirty years. She is also a Certified Aveda Colorist and enjoys continuing her education on natural hair maintenance and overall hair health via local and national classes throughout each year.

After opening her own salon in 2010, her clientele grew exponentially in just one year allowing her to see record numbers. Her current Smyrna, GA hair salon is just minutes from the new Braves stadium at SunTrust Park, Cumberland Mall, and Cobb Galleria.

Her multi-layered hair services meet all of her clientele's haircare needs with natural hair maintenance, gentle dimensional color, achieving their hair growth goals, extra-long hair care and maintenance, silkpress and thermal/temporary waving, permanent waving, smoothing treatments, bridal and special occasion styling, braiding, brows, lashes, and short/clipper cuts.

Her clients have nicknames for her which include, The Hair Doctor, the Hair Whisperer and has been cited for making even the most stubborn or difficult natural hair surrender to her "touch."

Meet Mo'.

What is the most common myth regarding natural haircare that you hear from your clients?

The most common myth regarding haircare that I hear from "natural hair" clients is the belief that "natural" hair is naturally stronger and since it has no chemical straightening or heat (or very little) it rarely needs a trim.

But don't let the natural coils fool you. Curly hair is naturally drier and more porous than straighter hair. It is affected by most everything around it, especially sun, pollutants, hard water, and indoor heating and air conditioning systems. Sometimes just using the wrong products (ingredients) or none at all can aid in dried-out, "crispier" ends.

Naturalistas should stay in tune with their hair strand's ends. When strand ends begin to:
- *Feel drier or harder than the rest of your hair shaft,*
- *Require more product to "moisturize" or perk them up,*
- *Have loosened or lost their "curl pattern,"*
- *"Mat up" easily,*
- *Are difficult to comb through...it's probably time for a trim!*

What are the top three tips you give to your clients regarding caring for their natural hair?

I tend to do a lot, I mean a ton, of sharing and explaining during an appointment. For example, I will talk in-depth about the product or products I might be using to style someone's hair, why I'm using it, and a few different ways my client can use it, while <u>demonstrating</u> how I am using it for that service.

My top three tips for natural haircare that I share most often are:

1) TRIM YOUR ENDS OFTEN!!!
Yes, that means quarterly. At least two to four times per year, not once in a while or yearly. Your perky ends and longer, stronger strands will thank you for stopping your "ends" from splitting and spreading up the hair shaft, with regular trims.

2) Sleep on a non-cotton pillowcase (silkier textures).
The absorbent cotton fibers act as a sponge on hair's ends (while you sleep), robbing moisture and forcing more frequent trimming of "dead", lifeless ends.

3) Essential oils are your hair's friend.
Find the one(s) that work best <u>for your hair</u>. Then apply spar-

ingly to your hair's "edges and ends," daily, after shampooing or as needed to protect against dryness and breakage. Also, boost your conditioning by adding oils to your final conditioning and/or to your "leave-in" conditioner.

Water-soluble (easily removed) silicones like cyclomethycaine and dimethicone copolyol are lightweight (non-oil) options for thinner hair. This note is for those wanting to avoid oils when wearing temporary, thermally "straightened" hairstyling. Silicones protect hair from heat and elements while keeping it smooth and shiny by "waterproofing" each strand. It gives hair slippage, allowing for less tangling and has conditioning benefits of sealing and locking in conditioner.

Monique Broussard
Hair We Geaux Salon
760 Concord Road SE, Smyrna, GA 30082
678.293.6200 - www.StyleSeat.com/i/moniqueperry

CHAPTER 9: NATURAL-HAIRED CHIRREN'

It starts in the developmental stages of a young person's life —during childhood. Confidence, that is. Whether you're the black parent of beautiful natural-haired babies and need reinforcement self-acceptance while instilling confidence about their natural hair, or if you're completely clueless about how to care for your child's natural tresses, or like me—without kids altogether but have young people in your life - breeding an environment of confidence when wearing natural hair is key. The language you communicate to your natural-haired babes while they're youngins is critical to their self-loving developmental phase.

Encourage Them to Experiment

The fun part about natural hair is that it's versatile and trainable. Buns, silk presses, locs, twist sets, braids, WnG's—there are so many options available to us in which our natural hair can be worn. Encouraging children at a young age while inspiring them to find their own version of beauty will allow your young ones to develop authentic confidence about what beauty looks like to them and how they like to wear their hair.

Up until age twelve, my mother would plait my hair into sections every one to two weeks and always on a Sunday. However, when it was picture time at school, special holidays, vacations and such, she'd style my hair in a different way. Pigtails, sometimes straightened; oh, but the little buns were cute too. I would become excited when she would do my hair because it was a time when we'd bond for at least an hour and a half. I think those plaiting hair sessions allowed our mother/daughter relationship to flourish as I approached my preteen years. In addition, I found joy in the process of her doing my hair because she would make positive remarks while doing it—even though in retrospect, I know she would be dead tired many evenings while trying to navigate my sometimes unruly kinks and coils.

Walk the Talk

Now, this one may rub some the wrong way, and that's okay. The bottom line is, monkey see, monkey do. Even if you never wear your natural hair, having images around the home, whether that be other family members with their natural hair, TV shows that have natural haired actors and actresses, or even if you personally wear your natural hair out all the time—perception is everything. It's all about showing children versatility while confidently wearing your natural hair.

Children need to see the message being portrayed to them in real life. Telling your child they have lovely natural hair while making negative comments toward another texture of hair on someone also doesn't help the cause. Let's be sure we don't accidentally instill discriminatory and post-slavery mentality ways of thinking in our young ones by putting some hair textures down over others. Let's educate our youth about their hair history and make them proud and empowered to wear their natural hair.

Till this day, I am still trying to perfect two styles my mom wore best on her beautiful hair: the WnG and the half up/half down, tousled look. As I'd watch her do her hair daily, she took much care in crafting the perfect slicked-back ponytails, low buns, and straight looks. I wanted to spend time on my hair the way she spent on hers. I wanted to be beautiful like my mother in the same way many little girls look at their mom—as someone they oftentimes aspire to be. Ensuring you are playing an intentional role with developing your child's perception on natural beauty is important to your child's development.

Men have a special ability to affect a young boy or girl's life. Dads, understanding how much weight your word has on your little ones' egos, confidence, and overall self-perception is crucial. It's important to say positive and encouraging words when speaking to your child about their hair, your hair, and frankly any natural-haired person. It's all about using positive language, proper natural hair education and examples when shaping the mind early on in an effort to encourage and empower our black youth.

Learn How to do Their Hair

If you have a child with difficult hair or mixed-race hair or if you're the Caucasian parent of a melanated child—you have no excuse to not have your child's hair healthy. No excuses. As mentioned earlier, taking the time to do your child's hair leads to bonding moments that are beneficial for parents and children alike. If you're just not able to twist, condition, braid, loc or maintain your child's hair on your own, find a trusted professional who can. It's important for melanated children to be able to take pride in their hair from a very young age. This positive outlook on their hair from a young age allows them to see themselves in a unique and beautiful light.

CHAPTER 10: RESHAPING OUR HAIR VIEW

So let's say you didn't grow up in an environment where natural hair was appreciated and definitely not celebrated. You want to think differently. But for whatever reason, you've had a difficult time with the way you see natural hair. I mean, you want to love it but you don't.

It's time to *reshape* your hair view—yea, pun intended. But how?

Learn Your *HAIRstory*

In the opener of this book, we did a light dive into African American *Hair*story here in this country. I encourage you to instigate more research on your own when it comes to our *Hair*story. The more educated you are about your history, the more your mind is available to accept changed mental perceptions.

Experiment with Different Styles & Products

Once you learn your *HAIRstory*, then you can start trying out styles on your hair that you've never tried before. I suggest finding a social media hair guru that is most closely relatable to your hair texture so you can visit their resources for backup as we talked about in Chapter 6. Sometimes, you'll find that the styles you thought you loved don't look as flattering on you as you imagined and the styles you didn't think you'd like probably look more amazing on you than you thought! The more styles you introduce into your natural hair regimen, the more excited you'll become when having to do your hair weekly or daily.

Do the BIG CHOP

I don't mean Big Chop in regards to cutting off relaxed portion of your hair. I mean, do the Big Chop when it comes to toxic, stinkin-thinkin'. Chop away at prejudice, discrimination, self-loathing and categorization of how natural hair is *supposed* to look. Why must melanated beauties of soft caramel tones not feel black enough because of their mixed ethnicity? Why must brown beauties be considered too dark to have beautiful hair? Oh, can we also kill the GOOD HAIR/BAD HAIR façade? Why should we continue to use language that was initially used to divide us in our everyday culture? We shouldn't. The theme for melanated naturals should be: Mobilization and Uplift. Let's be the example our kids needs from us. Let's be the cataclysmic change that turns culture's thinking around when it comes to Blacks and natural hair.

Find Other Naturals

Community is important in regard to any major movement, right? Whether you're trying to open a new business, dive deeper into your faith, or connect with other parents for tips—having a community is a difference-maker and is oftentimes the key to securing your knowledge in a given area. I encourage naturals (especially the ones just joining the movement) to attend natural hair conferences, festivals, and shows while connecting with other naturals who are looking for encouragement, support, and advice. There are so many groups of naturals—both men and women, on Facebook—that the networking opportunities with other naturals are endless!

Reconstruct Your Version of Beauty

Oftentimes, we may have a skewed view of how our natural hair looks due to years of unequal racial tactics that have been passed down since the beginning of slavery in the United States.

Together, we will refuse to allow the generational side-effects of divisive language to continue to negatively affect self-image in the black community surrounding hair. While you are attempting to reconstruct your version of what beautiful is, may you have grace on yourself while remembering the years of difficulty lived by *our* ancestors. Once you learn new styles that cater to your luscious natural locks, you can then begin to love *your* version of beauty.

I hope you feel empowered, educated, knowledgeable, and eager to adopt new or improved techniques to your natural hair care regimen. Natural Hair is just one thing I love to talk about; see all the other topics I discuss at LifestyleofMoore.com and be sure to subscribe while you're there!

NATURAL HAIR GLOSSARY

ACV - Apple Cider Vinegar

A beneficial treatment for natural, kinky and curly hair. A Natural scalp has a pH of -5. ACV has a natural pH of 3 but when diluted, its pH level more closely matches the natural scalp. Balancing the pH of our hair is important for the overall root health of the strands helping to prevent hair loss and breakage. Using ACV as a final rinse will result in: the hair being shinier and less frizzy. Oftentimes, the underlying cause of hair loss and dandruff is bacteria. Since ACV is an anti-inflammatory and antifungal treatment, naturals can find benefits in multiple areas.

Afro

A hairstyle made popular during the 1960s amongst members of the Black Panther Party that includes tight coils or curls coiffed around the head.

AWS (Andre Walker System)

The classification of defining hair texture as created by Andre Walker, Oprah Winfrey's hairstylist. Straight (1), wavy (2), curly (3) or kinky (4). Personally, I'm a 3A-3B. Knowing your hair type is one way to create an optimal hair regimen that's specific to your hair.

Banding

Method used to stretch the hair by using ponytail holders or hair ties to stretch natural hair in place while it is drying.

Bantu Knots
Actual term: Zulu knots. This is when the hair is sectioned off into a square or diamond-like pattern and the hair is twisted around in knots.

BC (Big Chop)
The act of completely cutting off chemically treated hair leaving only natural strands behind.

BJCO (Black Jamaican Castor Oil)
Due to being cold-pressed, natural castor oil retains many of its nutrients and fatty acids. Pure castor oil is filled with Omega 9 and Omega 6 fatty acids and has many antifungal/ antibacterial agents within its makeup that assist with less hair breakage and more hair growth.

Braid and Curl
A style that is created after the hair is braided in typically larger sections with a curl-defining tool at the end of each braid (a flexi-rod or roller, etc.) and then taken apart. This still can be done on dampened or moist hair and will typically reveal a more defined curled style.

Brazilian Keratin Treatment
A method by which you temporarily straighten the hair without using harsh chemicals.

Comb Coil
A style that involves taking the end of a rattail comb and twisting the hair around the comb in a clockwise fashion. This can be worn as a protective style and is great for shorter hair lengths.

Co-Wash
Cleansing the hair with conditioner instead of shampoo.

Creamy Crack
A term created by women of color that describes how diffi-

cult it is to stop using Permanents, which are typically white and creamy in texture, to straighten their hair.

DC (Deep Conditioning)

The process of adding a conditioner to your hair for an extended period of time in addition to including a heat source for optimal penetration of the conditioner. This process is known to add moisture back to dry strands.

Denman Brush

A styling tool that detangles with 5-7 rows of bristles that are ideal for evening product throughout hair, detangling and defining curls.

Dusting

The method of trimming less than ¼ inches of hair. The discarded hair resembles dust and is significantly less hair trimmed than a traditional trim.

Ends

A reference given to the oldest part of the hair shaft—the very bottom or "ends."

EVCO (Extra Virgin Coconut Oil)

Ensuring the coconut oil is cold-press/extra-virgin and is being sold in a glass jar is pertinent. As I expressed earlier, EVCO is my hair's favorite, so I always have at least one jar of fresh EVCO on hand at any given time. EVCO is packed with Vitamin E so it's an amazing sealant of moisturizing after dampening the hair.

EVOO (Extra Virgin Olive Oil)

Many naturals use this oil as a moisturizer for hair. It's important to purchase high-quality olive oil from a glass jar. You can find this on your neighborhood grocery aisle. It's also a great source for skin moisture as well. The glass jar helps keep the oil's exposure to sunlight and oxygen to a minimum, which can cause the oil to become rancid.

Twist-Set/Out

A style that involves double stranding the hair to the scalp to create a twist that is flat to the head like cornrows. A flat twist style can be done on dry or wet hair. The twists are then unraveled to create a uniformed curl pattern throughout.

FSG (Flax Seed Gel)

A natural product created by boiling and straining the flax seeds that creates a gel to be refrigerated and used on the hair. This gel adds moisture to the hair and has amazing slip which is ideal for braided or twisted styles. You can make flaxseed gel even more moisturizing by adding some of your favorite hair oil to the gel.

Fluff

The method of creating more volume and fullness using a comb by lifting the roots or your fingers to separate the curls.

LOC Method

Method by which liquid, oil and conditioner are used [and in that order] to moisturize hair.

No-poo

Method of cleansing the hair without using shampoo (i.e. see Co-wash and ACV).

Pineapple

A method of preserving natural hairstyles, especially twist-outs and curls, by piling hair on top of head in a loosely secured ponytail or silk scarf.

Pre-Poo

The process by which conditioner is applied to the hair prior to cleansing with shampoo. This can aid in the moisture and detangling process.

Product Junkie

Slang used for a person who purchases product after product looking for the next hottest thing on the market.

Protective Style
A method of wearing natural hair which prevents frequent manipulation leading to the promotion of hair growth.

Sealing
The method of locking moisture into the hair by dampening with water and proceeding with the LOC method (see LOC).

SilkPress
A way of pressing the hair in which it looks like it has been relaxed using a high-quality flat iron. It does not involve a hot comb like the original press-n-curl.

Slip
The description often used in regards to conditioner or a detangler that easily detangles hair allowing it to "slip" through your fingers or comb.

Sisterlocks
Locs that are about half the size of traditional locs. Proper research on a Certified Sisterlock consultant should be done because improper installation can lead to hair loss.

SLS - Sodium Lauryl Sulfate
A foaming agent used in many beauty products such as shampoo which can cause drying to natural hair.

Transitioning
Term used to describe someone who is going through the process of growing out their chemically processed hair.

Virgin Hair
Natural hair that has never received any chemical treatments (permanents, color, etc.).

Wash Day

Slang that naturals use to describe the one day that's dedicated to natural hair care. My wash day is Sunday. When is yours?

WnG (Wash and Go)

A style used to wear natural hair by way of washing with conditioner and applying a styling product such as gel or styling cream. Style can be completed by air-drying or a diffuser.

ABOUT THE AUTHOR

Ashley is a Georgia-born natural hair enthusiast, model, blogger and corporate professional who has been on her own natural hair journey for the last 10 years. In addition to being passionate about survivors of domestic violence and working for a top Medical Technology company, Ashley feels strongly about educating people of color on their hair and encouraging them to feel beautiful in their natural state. She has earned several personal, professional and philanthropic accomplishments over the last 3 years including Georgia State University's *40 Under 40 for 2018* as well as a *Sales Impact Award* from National Sales Network – Atlanta Chapter. As a lover of literature, in 2019, Ashley decided to launch her personal writings on LifestyleofMoore.com, a lifestyle blog that focuses on food, travel and worldly life perspectives. Ashley currently lives in Las Vegas, Nevada.

Made in the USA
Las Vegas, NV
23 April 2022

47913060R00038